Irritable Bowel Syndrome

Natural and Herbal Remedies to Cure Irritable Bowel Syndrome

K.M. KASSI

© Copyright 2014 by _____K.M. KASSI_____ All rights reserved.

This document is geared towards providing exact and reliable information in regards to the topic and issue covered. The publication is sold with the idea that the publisher is not required to render accounting, officially permitted, or otherwise, qualified services. If advice is necessary, legal or professional, a practiced individual in the profession should be ordered.

- From a Declaration of Principles which was accepted and approved equally by a Committee of the American Bar Association and a Committee of Publishers and Associations.

In no way is it legal to reproduce, duplicate, or transmit any part of this document in either electronic means or in printed format. Recording of this publication is strictly prohibited and any storage of this document is not allowed unless with written permission from the publisher. All rights reserved.

The information provided herein is stated to be truthful and consistent, in that any liability, in terms of inattention or otherwise, by any usage or abuse of any policies, processes, or directions contained within is the solitary and utter responsibility of the recipient reader. Under no circumstances will any legal responsibility or blame be held against the publisher for any reparation, damages, or monetary loss due to the information herein, either directly or indirectly.

Respective authors own all copyrights not held by the publisher.

The information herein is offered for informational purposes solely, and is universal as so. The presentation of the information is without contract or any type of guarantee assurance.

The trademarks that are used are without any consent, and the publication of the trademark is without permission or backing by the trademark owner. All trademarks and brands within this book are for clarifying purposes only and are the owned by the owners themselves, not affiliated with this document.

TABLE OF CONTENTS

Introduction 1

Chapter 1 : Irritable Bowel Syndrome: An Overview 2

Chapter 2 : Laboratory Tests & Diagnostic Procedures to
      Determine Irritable Bowel Syndrome 5

Chapter 3: Natural Remedies for IBS 10

Chapter 4 : Herbal Remedies to Combat IBS 18

Chapter 5 : Other Alternative Therapies for IBS 23

Chapter 6 : Living a Fulfilled Life Even with IBS 28

Conclusion 30

Introduction

I want to thank you and congratulate you for downloading the book, *"Irritable Bowel Syndrome: Natural and Herbal Remedies to Cure Irritable Bowel Syndrome"*.

This book contains proven steps and strategies on how to manage Irritable Bowel Syndrome or IBS and prevent it from controlling your life.

IBS afflicts millions of people worldwide. The symptoms range from mild to severe; albeit, the long-term effects are the same – a decrease in the quality of life.

There are many medicines that are believed to be effective in alleviating the symptoms of IBS. However, these medicines have adverse outcomes that can affect the quality of life of the afflicted person. Is there another effective way to manage IBS without the negative effects?

The good news is there is! There are natural and herbal remedies to help an IBS sufferer overcome chronic symptoms of this medical condition. These practical remedies are guaranteed to work. Plus, they are easy to do and affordable.

You may have an IBS, but you can still have that rewarding, fulfilling, successful life that you dream of. Find out the truth about IBS and be free from its hold starting today.

Thanks again for downloading this book, I hope you enjoy it!

Chapter 1

Irritable Bowel Syndrome: An Overview

Irritable bowel syndrome or IBS is considered as the most prevalent functional gastrointestinal disorder worldwide. In US alone, there are around 25-45 millions of people with IBS, mostly females. Even children are afflicted with IBS.

What does functional GI disorders mean? It is having a dysfunctional but seemingly normal gastrointestinal system. There are no structural or biochemical abnormalities of the organs that are seen on diagnostic tests yet there are symptoms indicating the presence of a problem. In short, the problem itself is the motility (movement) of the digestive system and not any damage to its tissues.

Symptoms vary from person to person. Some are mild and tolerable while others are severe and debilitating.

Some of the symptoms include:
- Gas
- A bloated feeling
- Abdominal pain or cramping
- Constipation or diarrhea or alternate bouts of the two
- Mucus in the stool
- Food intolerances
- Nausea

These symptoms are often relieved by bowel elimination. They seem simple and manageable. However, looking at them closely, one can see how they can alter the social and physical activities of the person and can limit what he can achieve in his life. Take the case of diarrhea. Imagine a guy talking to a client when diarrhea strikes. He would have no choice but to excuse himself. That incident may cause him to lose the opportunity to sell or close a deal.

How about a woman who is enjoying a date when all of a sudden, she experiences abdominal pain or cramping? That will ruin a good date and worse, a good relationship. Therefore, it is vital to halt these symptoms, so that one can live and enjoy a normal life.

A diagnosis of IBS can be concluded when:

- ➤ The symptoms last for more than 6 months.
- ➤ There are symptoms present for at least three times in a month.

How can IBS be acquired?

The exact cause of IBS remains a mystery to all. However, studies revealed that symptoms of IBS seem to result from disturbed interaction in the brain, gut and nervous system. What happens among these three?

A quick review of the anatomy and physiology of the bowels or intestines would help. Remember that the walls of intestines have layers of muscles that alternately contract and relax in a rhythm, causing the movement of food from stomach to intestinal tract until it reaches the rectum.

With IBS, these contractions can either be too strong (leading to the development of gas diarrhea and bloating) or too weak (leading to the slowed passage of food; hence, resulting to constipation).

What happened to the contractions? As the brain relays the message to the intestines to contract, somehow, the body mixes up the message and performs the inaccurate response – contractions that are either too strong or too weak. Why this occurs is still unsolved at this time.

There are "trigger points" that are considered to cause the symptoms to manifest, however. Here are some of them.

- Food. Studies show that certain foods can cause severe symptoms to appear to patients with IBS. Examples are cauliflower, milk, beans, cabbage, fats, chocolates, spices, alcohol and carbonated drinks.

- Stress. Events leading to heightened stress such as a major exam or new job have been implicated as among the major causes, too.

- Hormones. More women are afflicted with IBS and the probable cause is hormones. Documented reports of symptoms becoming worse before or during their menstrual period led to this conclusion.

- Other illnesses. Stomach illnesses like gastroenteritis or bacterial overgrowth can also trigger IBS. These illnesses can lead to changes in normal bowel movement.

- Psychological conditions such as depression or anxiety also produce the symptoms of IBS.

IBS is a chronic disorder where symptoms can worsen or improve. These signs signal that IBS is getting worse: there is bleeding in the rectum and progressive or nocturnal (appears at night) abdominal pain. Plus, there is weight loss.

On the other hand, symptoms can improve to the point as if they have disappeared completely. They would occasionally be experienced once in a while but that would be about it. There is no major impact to the person at all.

The primary cause of IBS may be a mystery but its solution has been established; therefore, the person can go on and have a normal life despite being diagnosed with IBS. The next chapter will discuss who are at risk for IBS and what are the laboratory and diagnostic exams needed to determine IBS. Read on.

Chapter 2

Laboratory Tests & Diagnostic Procedures to Determine Irritable Bowel Syndrome

A person with no previous signs and symptoms of Irritable Bowel Syndrome may suddenly experience them. Why is this so? Who are most likely to develop the condition? Here are some factors that may increase the risk of some people and acquire IBS in the process:

- **Gender** - Women are found to be 2 times more likely to develop the condition than men. Hormonal reasons are being attributed to this.

- **Age** - People aged 25-45 are more at risk than others. The possible reason for this is because of heightened stress at this stage. It is at this age that a person builds his career, starts his family and works his way to making all his dreams come true. In short, it is the most stressful time of his life. Although stress is not named as one of the causes of IBS, it is directly linked to the manifestations of signs and symptoms.

- **Genetic disposition** - Although still lacking in evidences and further study, a relationship between genes and IBS is being considered as a risk factor.

- **With mental illnesses**. Anxiety, depression, sexual and physical abuses make the person more susceptible to acquire IBS. This may be related to stress, effects to the brain of these conditions or alteration in the diet as caused by these illnesses.

As early as possible, the person should seek a medical professional help to combat IBS. If left untreated, this medical condition can lead to the following complications:

- ➢ **Malnourished state.** Food intolerances, bloating, gas, nausea, diarrhea, and abdominal cramping can reduce the food intake of the person. The needed nutrients and calories of the body are not met.

- ➢ **Hemorrhoids.** Alternate bouts of diarrhea and constipation can lead to the development of hemorrhoids.

- ➢ **Effect to the quality of life of the person**. The worst complication is being unable to live life the fullest. This can lead to discouragement and depression to the person, further aggravating the situation.

IBS has signs and symptoms that are similar to other medical conditions. One example is celiac disease. The person with celiac disease has sensitivity to barley, rye and wheat. Their symptoms match those of IBS.

To confirm the diagnosis of IBS, the doctor will do a thorough physical assessment and research about the medical history of the patient. At the same time, he will suggest the following laboratory tests to be taken. These are:

Routine blood test - This will help determine the health status of the person, whether he is well or ill. At the same time, it can reveal the presence of foreign bodies or microorganisms when the white blood cells are elevated.

Stool exams - With chronic diarrhea, the doctor will assess for bacteria or parasites in the stool. Also, the stools of those with lactose intolerance will be foamy and loose.

Breath test - Helicobacter pylori (H. pylori) refers to bacteria that infect the stomach and intestine of the person. It is the causative factor of gastritis, gastric or duodenal ulcers and eventually, gastric cancer. In this test, the doctor will get a sample of the person's breath and check for the presence of this bacteria.

This exam is useful in checking for lactose intolerance. On the day of the exam, the person will be asked to consume a liquid with lactose then breath samples will be taken. If high levels of hydrogen were found, that could be indicative of lactose intolerance.

Lactose intolerance test - Again, the person will be asked to drink a liquid with lactose on it. Afterwards, his blood sugar level will be checked every 30 minutes for 2 hours. Positive results will yield low blood sugar level.

Diagnostic Exams to assess IBS

Further tests may be required to conclude the diagnosis of IBS. Here are some of them:

Routine X-Ray - This is just to check the structure of the vital organs. Usually, this will yield a negative result. As explained, there is usually nothing wrong with the organs themselves. It is their function that is faulty.

Colonoscopy - This is necessary to check the inner lining and total condition of the entire length of the colon. A small flexible tube (called colonoscope) will be inserted into the colon through the anus. At the end of the tube is a camera, allowing the doctor to see and inspect the colon and its surrounding. Colonoscopy can help the doctor see the following:

- Colon polyps
- Ulcers
- Tumors
- Areas of inflammation
- Bleeding

Computed tomography colonography (CTC scan) - This is a cross section imaging of the colon. This will allow a better view and detail of the organ, tissue or blood vessels of the colon. It is a non-invasive, painless procedure. The patient will be asked to lie down on the machine, which has a tunnel-like feature. Images will be taken while he is lying on his back, on his stomach and on his side.

Flexible sigmoidoscopy - This is basically the same as colonoscopy, only the lower part of the colon would be seen and not its entire length. As with colonoscopy, a small tube will be inserted in the sigmoid through the anus. The sigmoid, rectum and surrounding areas will also be examined for any abnormality.

Lower GI series – is also known as barium enema - This is the use of barium sulfate (dye) to detect abnormalities in the colon. The dye will be injected in the colon via the anus and that will outline the whole large intestine. Any defect or abnormality will be seen through the monitor.

The problem with IBS is that the symptoms can be tolerated; hence, seldom do patients seek medical help. They just buy over-the-counter drugs to manage pain, diarrhea, constipation and other symptoms of IBS. This causes the condition to progress in terms of its severity without the knowledge of the patient. At the end, the condition would have worsened and it would be more difficult to manage it already.

Therefore, one should be alert for any alteration in the body systems. These are clues regarding the status and overall health of the person. Early detection is vital to early diagnosis and management. Also, there is better prognosis when early management is done.

The experts use 2 tests to determine the existence of IBS. First is called the Rome criteria. In here, the qualified person is one who has reported abdominal pain for at least three days in a month for 3 months. In addition, the following symptoms are also present: alteration in frequency, pattern and consistency of stools. Plus, there is feeling of being bloated and the passage of mucus.

The second one is the Manning criteria. Patients who have complained of the following symptoms are diagnosed with IBS:
- At the beginning of abdominal pain, there is loose stool
- Abdominal pain being relieved by defecation
- May complain of incomplete bowel movement, changes in the stool
- With more frequent bowel movement
- Mucus in stool
- Visible distention

IBS is not easy to diagnose, as the symptoms appear to be very general. However, when the person seeks early consultation, the probability of accurate diagnosis is higher plus the prognosis of the condition is better.

As soon as diagnosis of IBS is confirmed, the person should start focusing on management and treatment. There are many ways to control IBS. The succeeding chapters are the guidelines to painless, symptoms-free, natural and herbal remedies to IBS.

Chapter 3:

Natural Remedies for IBS

Pharmacological management is common among IBS patients. Doctors usually prescribe drugs that can alleviate the symptoms of IBS. There are specific drugs that are believed to be the cure for IBS. However, these drugs are found to have adverse side effects, too. Some of the side effects of these drugs include:

- Headache
- Nausea
- Stomach upset
- Diarrhea
- Constipation
- Distention or bloating
- Difficulty in urinating
- Drowsiness
- Depression

As one will notice, the side effects are mostly gastrointestinal-related also. Therefore, instead of really helping relieve the symptom, they are sometimes causing more problems for the person; hence, natural remedies will be the better option.

Prerequisites

> As with all procedures, the primary health care provider should be informed and updated even of the intention to follow natural and herbal remedies. It should be done with the knowledge and approval of the doctor.

- ➤ Also, if there is a need to treat existing medical condition related to IBS, for example, intestinal bacterial growth, it is a must to deal with this first. The doctor usually orders antibiotics to eradicate these bacteria. Afterwards, natural remedies can be started.

- ➤ Remember, knowledge is power. Therefore, it is the responsibility of the person to get as much information as he can about IBS. The more he knows about his enemy, the better he can prepare in dealing with it.

What are the things he can do to increase his awareness about IBS?

- Check online and offline information about IBS.
- Ask his physician about it.
- Interview other patients diagnosed with IBS (if possible).
- Join a support group of IBS patients.
- Volunteer to assist patients with IBS (if possible only).

Why choose the natural remedies over the pharmacological therapy?

Here are some advantages of natural remedies:

1. Effectiveness. These remedies will also produce the same effects as the drugs sans the discomfort and side effects.

2. Value for money. Most of the remedies are free of charge plus they can result to more savings. For instance, there is no money involved in trying to cease from a bad habit like smoking. On the contrary, one gets to save a lot of money from not buying cigarettes, not getting sick because of cigarettes and feeling better with the absence of the habit.

3. Easy to do. There may be some minor adjustments (on lifestyle modification) but the remedies are easy and fun to do.

4. Healthier to the body. There are no known negative effects of using these natural remedies. Instead, there is guarantee of better health, not only in relation to IBS, but also to the general condition and wellbeing of the person.

What are these natural remedies?

Change in diet

Diet plays a major role in "triggering" the symptoms of IBS to manifest. Therefore, it is also the answer in making sure that the symptoms will not be experienced. Here are some things to avoid:

- Gluten. It is found in rye, barley and wheat; therefore, any products made from these grains have gluten in them and should be avoided too. These are the products to avoid. They include but not limited to the following:
    - Wheat flour
    - Graham flour
    - Whole wheat flour
    - Wheat germ
    - Wheat bran
    - Foods made with wheat may include:
        - Pasta
        - Bread
        - Cookies
        - Pastries
        - Muffins
        - Cereals
        - Cakes
        - Crackers
        - Beer
        - Oats
        - Dressing

Note: Before one reacts how difficult this is (after all, these are foods that most people love to eat), take note that there are available gluten-free products similar to the list. Hence, the IBS sufferer should simply replace the ingredients with gluten-free ones to prepare these favorite items.

Take note also that one will benefit not only from being free of IBS symptoms but also from the development of other medical conditions such as diabetes and its complications.

- Gas-forming foods. Passing gas is normal albeit embarrassing. With IBS patients however, abdominal gases can lead to pain and distention. In order to avoid the discomfort of gas, one should avoid these gas-producing foods:
  - Vegetables such as asparagus, brussel sprouts, cabbage, green peppers, cucumbers, peas, raw potatoes, broccoli, radishes, and artichokes.
  - Fruits such as bananas, melon, prunes, raw apples, peaches, and apricots.
  - Beans and legumes.
  - Eggs
  - Fried and fatty foods.
  - Carbonated drinks.
  - Sugar and sugar substitutes.
  - Foods with lactose.
  - Milk and other dairy products.
- Avoid caffeine – this can promote diarrhea. At the same time, it can hamper the sleeping pattern of the person. Adequate rest and sleep is essential for managing the symptoms of IBS.

- Avoid spicy foods. They contain capsaicin, which can cause spasm of the large intestine, leading to diarrhea.

- Stay away from FODMAPS. This stands for Fermentable Oligosaccharides, Disaccharides, Monosaccharides And Polyols. These foods cannot be completely digested in the stomach and they attract intestinal bacteria. The foods to avoid are those high in fructancs, fructose, lactose, polyols and galactans. Examples are:
    - Garlic
    - Onions
    - Celery
    - Mushrooms
    - Taro
    - Blackberries
    - Dates
    - Figs
    - Lychee
    - Mangoes
    - Raisins
    - Watermelon
    - Processed meats
    - Condiments, sauces, dips and sweeteners
    - Some beverages
    - Dairy foods

What foods and drinks to take?

Experiment with fiber – As mentioned, diarrhea is one of the symptoms of IBS. Therefore, one should consume high fiber foods accordingly. When the symptoms of diarrhea appear, change to low fiber diet.

Probiotics – these are the "good bacteria" that one must consume for they help control the growth of the harmful bacteria, specifically in the intestines. Among the best sources of probiotics are yogurt, miso soup, soft cheeses, sourdough bread and sauerkraut.

Prebiotics – these are carbohydrates, which cannot be digested by the body. They serve as food for probiotics. They also help maintain a healthy digestive system. Examples are Jerusalem Artichokes, oatmeal, legumes, bananas and asparagus.

Water - Drinking 8 glasses or more of water helps in many ways. It can relieve constipation, for one. When there is diarrhea, on the other hand, it can prevent fluid imbalances due to fluid loss.

Drink peppermint tea – Peppermint has been used as a cure for indigestion for thousands of years already. The main active ingredients that make peppermint effective as an anti-spasmodic agent are menthol and methyl salicylate. They can produce the calming effects on the muscular layer of the stomach and intestine, including the uterus.

Peppermint tea is also known as a powerful analgesic. It provides relief from pain by blocking the pain signal transmission. At the same time, it can relieve, cramps, gas, morning sickness and bloated feeling. Fresh or dried peppermint with water can be brewed and taken as hot tea.

Other tips include not skipping meals. Instead, eat small, frequent meals. This will avoid bloating and abdominal cramps.

Do regular exercise

Aside from diet, physical activities are noted to help reduce the symptoms of IBS. Exercise can improve the circulation of the body; hence, oxygenated blood is delivered to all vital organs and body parts. At the same time, exercise makes the muscles strong especially on the abdominal area. The contraction and relaxation of the muscular layers of the intestines usually improve with exercise. Regular exercise is highly recommended for those with IBS.

Manage stress

Stress can trigger the symptoms of IBS. At the same time, when left untreated, it can further aggravate the symptoms of IBS and lead to complications, which will be more stressful to the person. Managing stress is therefore vital in keeping IBS under control.

What can be done?

1. Identify the stressors. These are the things, people, events, or places that are causing the stress. This could vary among people. For example, some people are easily irritated (stressed out) with traffic. This irritation can continue until they reach the office. It can affect their work and relationship with other people. Going home, traffic may be experienced also. Again, this can trigger stress. This time, it will be his family that would be affected with his irritation.

Others find it relaxing to be in a traffic jam for this is their time to meditate or pray; therefore, there are no negative emotions that are accumulated. They come to work refreshed and ready for challenges. How one faces the stressor will determine whether he will come out as a victor or victim of the situation. Therefore, when the person realizes what his stressors are, he can readily face them when they do come.

2. Identify his coping mechanisms. There are many defense mechanisms that one can utilize. He should find out which is the most suitable for him and try to adjust his coping mechanism with that.
3. Do the following relaxation techniques.
    a. Deep breathing exercise
    b. Massage
    c. Positive self talk
    d. Visualization

4. Communicate with other people. Be with friends. Go out and have a walk. Laugh out loud. Being with family or friends can help reduce stress.

5. Confess positive things. Instead of declaring negative things (that can only add to one's gloomy situation already), say sentences like "It's going to be okay" or "I can handle this".

These three natural remedies can do wonders for one's IBS already. Include other healthy lifestyles such as sleeping and resting for at least 8 hours a day, maintaining the ideal body weight and staying away from vices (cigarettes, alcohol, drugs), to name a few. These things are really beneficial to the person, not only in controlling their IBS symptoms, but more importantly, in keeping them healthy in all aspects of their life..

Chapter 4

Herbal Remedies to Combat IBS

The power of herbs is often overlooked in treating IBS. With these simple looking plants and herbs, it is actually possible to manage this condition. Here are some of the herbs that one can use to fight the symptoms of IBS and keep them away forever.

Peppermint – is named as the "drug of first choice" against IBS. It is known as a natural antispasmodic. It relaxes the smooth muscles of stomach and intestines, leaving a calm, numbing effect in the gastrointestinal tract. As the GI tract is calm, gas passes naturally; therefore, there is no abdominal pain, too.

Peppermint is believed to enhance gastric emptying. This means that foods do not stay longer than necessary in the stomach. It transfers to the small intestine as soon as it is ready for absorption. Delayed gastric emptying causes pain, discomfort and feeling of being bloated.

Peppermint contains essential oils that help stimulate the gallbladder to secrete bile, which is being used by the body to digest fats; hence, it is possible to prevent bloating with peppermint. Also, it can relieve one of diarrhea. One can use it as a tea (as discussed earlier) or eat it fresh, usually after a meal.

Other Uses of peppermint

Aside from its power to overcome gastrointestinal symptoms, peppermint is popular because of the following benefits:
- Helps lessen inflammation of the respiratory system to those with tuberculosis
- Controls allergic rhinitis by inhibiting the release of histamine

- Shingles-associated pain is reduced with topical application of peppermint oil
- Improves memory. By simply inhaling the aroma of peppermint, reports of increased alertness and better memory are given.
- Peppermint oil also relieves one of chemotherapy-induced nausea.
- It is very popular for dental use too. It whitens the teeth, freshen the breath and prevents cavities.
- Effective as a nasal decongestant and as a cough expectorant
- Helps relieve the pain from tension headache, too
- It has a stress-relieving aroma that soothes the nerves and calms the person.
- It is great for hair and skin health also.
- Used for asthma and muscle pains, too

Ginger – this is a light brown root with a distinctive taste. It contains high levels of magnesium, Vitamin C and other minerals. It is effective in providing the following benefits against IBS:

- Relieves nausea – In fact, during ancient time, travelers used this to overcome motion sickness.
- Improves stomach performance - Improves digestion and increases absorption of food. It is also known to relieve bloating and belching.
- Enhances appetite – Health is regained as the desire to take in food improves.
- Relieves stress – The strong aroma plus healing properties of ginger are believed to be the reasons for providing stress relief, so you can expect it to be helpful in avoiding and relieving IBS symptoms, too.

It may surprise a number of people to learn that ginger is not for IBS sufferers only but for everyone who desires to be healthy. Here are its other functions not related to gastrointestinal system:

- Reduce Inflammation – prevents hundreds of inflammatory diseases. At the same time, it can be applied topically to relieve one from physical inflammation of joints and muscles.
- Great in fighting respiratory problems – common coughs and environmental allergies are easily remedied with ginger.
- Improve blood circulation – which is equivalent to healthy organs and therefore, healthy systems.
- Relieve menstrual discomfort – cramps during one's period can be alleviated in two ways with ginger. First, boil the ginger with water. Use the concoction to soak a towel. Place the towel on the abdomen. Another method is to make a tea out of ginger. Add honey for a more delicious taste. Drink warm. Both methods are found effective in relieving menstrual discomfort.
- Increases fertility – Ancient doctors believed that ginger can solve erectile disorder. Also, it can help increase a male's sperm count.
- Others benefits include fighting off bacteria in the mouth and bad breath, detoxifying the liver, preventing cancer cells to proliferate and improving cholesterol levels.

Fennel – is effective for IBS treatment as it does the following:

- As an antispasmodic, it relaxes the lining of the entire gastrointestinal system.
- Its carminative property prevents gases from forming. It helps in the expulsion of gases, too.
- Gastric juices are produced through the stimulation of fennel. This aids in digesting the food easily, preventing bloating and indigestion.

- Other digestive problems such as stomachaches and cramps are relieved with this herb. How? It aids in regulating the contraction of the muscles in the intestinal wall.

Fennel seeds can be brewed to make a tea. Simply crush the seeds and add to a cup of hot water. Other people prefer chewing the seeds instead.

Fennel is used for other medical conditions such as respiratory tract infections, bronchitis, backache, cholera, visual problems, and even bedwetting. Women use fennel to increase the flow of breast milk, enhance sex drive and regulate menstrual cycle. Ancient doctors used fennel as a poultice for snakebites.

Chamomile – It is anti-inflammatory plus it helps relax smooth muscles of the intestines. It can be made into tea. Warm the tea and take 2 to 3- cups daily. This is found effective to relieve cramps, spasms, bloating, gas and other digestive problems.

Chamomile is also known as anti-peptic, antifungal and antibacterial. It is also popular for its sedative properties; hence, it is mainly taken before sleeping time.

Other uses of chamomile:
- Treatment of colds
- For healing of wounds and abscesses
- Treatment of skin conditions such as diaper rash, psoriasis and eczema.

Licorice – IBS sufferers find relief in the following symptoms using licorice:
- Gas
- Bloating
- Protects the lining of the stomach
- Soothes the stomach

Licorice is used for the following also:
- Cough
- Bronchitis
- Sore throat
- Food poisoning
- Malaria
- Liver disorder
- Chronic fatigue syndrome
- Tuberculosis

Wild yam – It can provide quick relief on the following IBS symptoms:
- Spasm
- Inflammation of the lining of the intestinal tract
- Cramps

Wild yam is oftentimes recommended for those with UTI problems as it has anti-inflammatory and anti-diuretic effects. It is also the favorite choice of those with arthritis, rheumatism and joint and muscle pains.

The plant is rich in diosgenin, which has an effect in the hormone, estrogen. As discussed, more women are afflicted with IBD, probably because of hormonal issues. With the help of this herb, the hormones can be manipulated and not cause the symptoms of the condition. Nowadays, instead of estrogen therapy, wild yam is the one being used.

One can find other herbs that are extremely useful in reducing or eliminating the symptoms of IBS. Discover the wonders of cayenne pepper, kava kava, lemon balm, catnips, and other herbs. Ask the doctor and herbalist about them..

Chapter 5

Other Alternative Therapies for IBS

Both natural and herbal remedies are effective in suppressing the manifestations of the symptoms of IBS. However, there are more therapies that can be implemented that will further help IBS sufferers to obtain relief from the discomfort and pain of having the medical condition. These are all natural too and do not make use of any drugs. Here are some of them:

Relaxation response meditation

IBS can be triggered by stress. One effective way to avoid stress, relax the muscles and achieve peace and stillness during difficult times is through this process. Here are the steps in doing this:

1. Sit in a comfortable position. Remain silent.
2. Close the eyes. Do not be distracted with any thoughts.
3. Beginning from the feet going up to the face, deeply relax the muscles one by one.
4. Start the deep breathing technique. Breath through the nose. Hold the breath for 3-5 seconds. Gently release the breath through pursed lips. Repeat the exercise. Be focused and aware of the breathing. To help maintain the concentration on breathing, say a meaningless word (example "one)) for each breath. When other distracting thoughts come, just continue focusing on breathing and on the chosen word. Breaths should not be forced but should be natural and effortless.
5. Continue this for 10-20 minutes. One can look at the time once in a while. The use of alarm clock is not recommended as it can

break the stillness and calm of the surrounding. Stay seated for several minutes with eyes open.

6. Stand up. The exercise is finished.

This therapy can be done once or twice a day, preferably 3 hours after a meal. During the procedure, if deep relaxation level is not reached, do not worry. Just continue to be in a calm state. Relaxation will occur in such state.

Gut Directed Hypnotherapy

IBS is considered as a brain-gut dysfunction; hence, this therapy answers the problem as it focuses on the mind yet the body benefits.

Hypnosis is not the loss of consciousness. Rather, it is re-directing the consciousness of the person from the distracting world to the peaceful internal processes.

Most people enjoy the relaxing, pleasant and comfortable feeling of being hypnotized. In the hypnotic state, the mind is open to positive thoughts and healing. Therefore, solutions to IBS symptoms are directed to the subconscious mind while in the state of complete rest.

Many physicians prescribe gut directed hypnotherapy for patients who did not achieve success with other conventional treatments of IBS. The effects of this therapy include:

- Reduction or relief from stress
- Can alleviate pain of all types and degrees

How is this done? A therapist will coax the IBS sufferer to a state of deep relaxation. While in this state, a program of suggestions will be processed. The patient is in full control of what action he would like to take. For example, he can fully visualize his digestive system to work perfectly, or he may be asked to place a hand over his abdomen and imagine a healing warmth flowing from the hand to the abdomen.

Although the actual mechanism of how hypnotherapy works remains a mystery, its effectiveness to treat all IBS symptoms cannot be denied. With this therapy, one may be diagnosed with the condition but no symptoms would be present. Hence, one can be considered as IBS-free.

Cognitive Behavioral Therapy

This therapy aims to shift the IBS patient's negative and stressful thoughts, behaviors and feeling into something positive and therapeutic by applying self-exploration exercises and other stress reducing strategies.

For example, upon interview, the doctor discovered that IBS symptoms of a patient are manifesting every time exam period is near. In order to reverse the situation, the person is asked to think of ways not to be stressed with exams. One action is doing advanced study. Or, conditioning of the mind can work, too. In here, the patient will "change his mind" regarding exams. Instead of looking at them as something negative, he would consider them as his way of showing to his teachers and parents that he had studied his lessons.

This therapy may take time to perfect but at the end, the benefits far outweigh the efforts poured into this.

Acupuncture

This therapy can offer relief for the abdominal pains experienced by IBS patients. The acupuncture needles are believed to stimulate the electromagnetic signals in the body. These signals release the natural pain-killing chemicals of the body.

Yoga

It relaxes both the mind and the body. As mentioned, stress is a causative factor of IBS. Yoga helps reduce or remove stress. At the same time, it promotes deep breathing exercises; therefore, the focus of the patient is shifted from the symptoms into his breathing.

There are 5 yoga poses that are known to relieve IBS symptoms. These are:

1. Parighasana or the gate pose. The patient assumes a tall kneeling position. He then attempts to stretch the right leg to the side, with the heel on the ground while the toes are reaching the floor. The, he should lift the left arm and lean the torso to the right. He must breathe properly. He should relax the face, mouth and jaw, as well.

2. Ardha matsyendrasana or the half-seated spinal twist. As named, the person is seated with his left leg extended and his right leg on top. Then he should slowly turn the torso towards the right leg. Breathe normally.

3. Jathara parivritti or reclining abdominal twist. Let the patient lie flat on his back. Then he should bend his right leg until it touches the belly. Hug the leg for a couple of seconds while breathing properly. Extend the right arm outside and let it touch the floor while the right leg continues to twist going to the left thigh and hip. Repeat this on the other side.

4. Salamba setu bandhasana or supported bridge pose. While lying flat on the back, just place a small pillow or blanket underneath the hip. Do deep breathing exercise and stay at this position for 5 minutes.

5. Ananda balasana or happy baby pose. Imagine the pose of a happy baby trying to reach his toes while on his back. The knees are bent while the hands are touching the big toes.

Warm baths can help, too. Add essential oils to the tub to relax and soothe the nerves. Soaking in bath while reading silently for 15 minutes can do the trick of relieving the person of stress; hence, relieving himself of IBS symptoms, too.

There are reports of massage, biofeedback technique and one-on-one counseling being effective in managing IBS, too. There are various studies being conducted to find more alternative methods to treat IBS.

Chapter 6

Living a Fulfilled Life Even with IBS

IBS can be debilitating, but with proper management and treatment, life can be made better. There are no preventions known that one can do to prevent the condition from affecting any individual but there are actions that can be taken to make it more bearable.

One important action is to be positive at all times. Someone who is optimistic sees the possibility of living a productive and fulfilling life even with IBS. Studies even confirmed that those who have positive perspective in life experiences the symptoms less frequently than those who are not. At the same time, even when symptoms do come, he can overcome them quickly.

A positive mental attitude is also a key in preventing stressors from getting the better out of the person. Even when the stressors are present, the person is not that affected. When stress is managed well, the symptoms are kept at bay, too.

Interestingly enough, those who are active in their spiritual life are found to be more in control of IBS. It can be attributed to the peace within. With their faith, they believe they have the ability to withstand the challenges of IBS. At the same time, they are more used to meditating, reflecting and relaxing, all of which are useful in controlling the symptoms of IBS.

IBS patients who are more sociable are also more capable of managing IBS symptoms. Social support, indeed, plays a major role in making IBS more tolerable. The patients are encouraged to spend more time with friends, family and even with new acquaintances and strangers. The more there is laughter, the lesser the pains and symptoms.

Finally, patients who do not focus on themselves realize that lesser symptoms of IBS occur. How to do this? Counting their other blessings is one way. Their physical health may not be that perfect but at least, they can still work, have a relationship and enjoy life in general. Instead of majoring or looking mostly on what they do not have, they should zoom in to what they are blessed with.

Volunteering to charity works is also a great way of shifting their focus away from themselves. Helping others make one more selfless. Also, most of the time, realization of how blessed they are compared with other people turn them into more positive individuals.

Lastly, finding people with IBS and helping them work in two ways. First, they learn more about the condition, which they would be able to use for themselves also. Second, they are able to help others cope up with the illness, too. That in itself is rewarding.

IBS need not be in charge of one's life. He can take over it. He can live with it. Most of all, he can enjoy a wonderful life even with IBS.

Conclusion

Thank you again for downloading this book!

I hope this book was able to help you understand Irritable Bowel Syndrome - its causes, risk factors, laboratory and diagnostic exams plus the natural and herbal remedies for it.

The next step is to have a productive, fulfilling life despite the diagnosis of IBS. It is possible to stop the symptoms of IBS from manifesting with the natural and herbal remedies mentioned in this book.

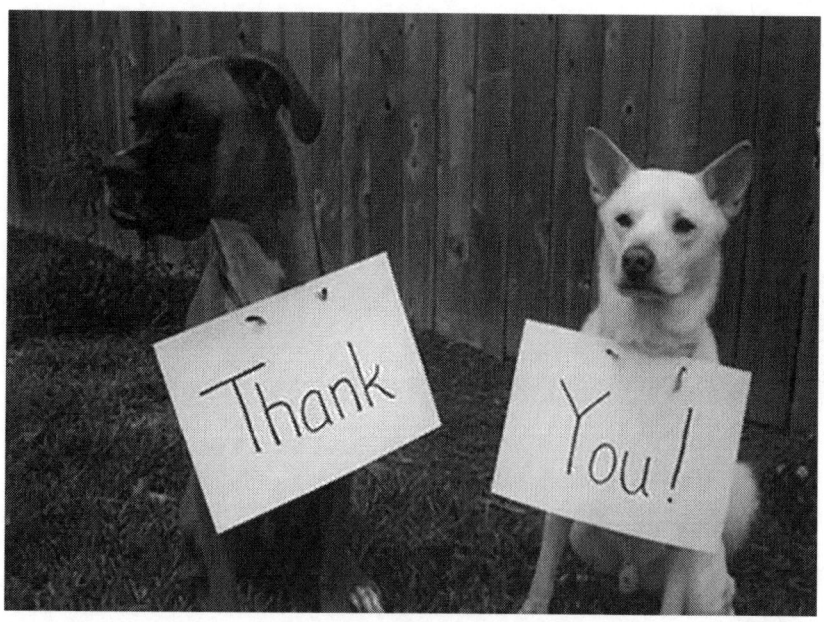

Finally, if you enjoyed this book, then I'd like to ask you for a favor, would you be kind enough to leave a review for this book on Amazon? It'd be greatly appreciated!

Click here to leave a review for this book on Amazon!

Made in the USA
Columbia, SC
06 May 2017